WEIGHT LOSS COOKBOOK AND GUIDE

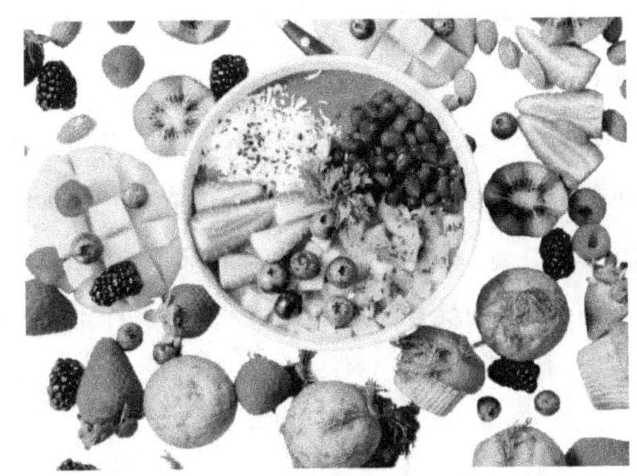

The Complete Guide and Recipes on How to Lose over 100 Pounds { With some tips and Tricks}.

SHEILA MAYNARD

Spinach and Feta Stuffed Chicken:

Grilled Vegetable Quesadillas:

Stuffed Bell Peppers with Quinoa and Chickpeas:

Mango Salsa Chicken:

Greek Chickpea Salad:

Shrimp and Broccoli Stir-Fry:

Mediterranean Quinoa Salad:

Panko-Crusted Baked Chicken Tenders::

Veggie Pita Sandwiches:

Lemon Herb Roasted Vegetables:

Thai Green Curry with Tofu:

Italian Sausage and Spinach Pasta:

Orange Glazed Salmon:

Lentil and Vegetable Soup:

Mushroom and Spinach Risotto:

Honey Garlic Baked Salmon:

Vegetarian Stuffed Bell Peppers:

Mango Avocado Salad:

Lemon Herb Grilled Shrimp:

Veggie Spring Rolls with Peanut Dipping Sauce:

Here are some tips and tricks to help you in your weight loss journey

CONCLUSION.

INTRODUCTION

In a quaint village nestled amidst rolling hills, lived a spirited individual named Emma. Known for her warm smile and boundless energy, Emma was on a personal journey to transform her life. Fueled by a desire to shed excess weight and embrace a healthier lifestyle, she embarked on a culinary adventure that would forever change her and the village's outlook on food.

As Emma navigated through farmers' markets, aromatic spice bazaars, and bustling kitchens, she uncovered the art of crafting flavors that not only tantalized the taste buds but also nourished the body. With each step of her journey, Emma discovered the power of mindful eating, balanced nutrition, and the joy of preparing meals that celebrated both health and indulgence.

Growing up in a household where food was a centerpiece of joy and togetherness, Emma's love for cooking was instilled at an early age. However, as the years went by, the pressures of modern life led her down a path of convenience foods and neglected self-care. That all changed one brisk morning when she took a long, hard look in the mirror, realizing that her reflection no longer mirrored the vibrant spirit she felt within.

With unwavering determination, Emma set out to transform her relationship with food. She immersed herself in books, consulted experts, and attended culinary workshops, each experience deepening her understanding of nutrition and its profound impact on well-being. Armed with newfound knowledge, she embarked on a mission to revitalize her village's culinary culture.

Word spread like wildfire throughout the village, as friends and neighbors eagerly sought Emma's guidance and recipes. The Weight Loss Cookbook and Guide was born out of Emma's passion and her commitment to helping others transform their lives through food. Within its pages, the secrets of Emma's journey were unveiled—recipes that made vegetables dance with vibrant colors, lean proteins sing with succulence, and whole grains weave stories of sustenance.

As Emma navigated the pages of her cookbook, she artfully wove personal anecdotes and insightful tips, making the journey not just about food but about embracing a holistic lifestyle change. She stressed the importance of finding balance, savoring each bite, and approaching wellness with compassion rather than rigidity.

Her story became an inspiration, a beacon of hope for those who had struggled with weight management and sought a realistic approach to healthier living. The once-dull kitchens of the village now echoed with laughter and the sizzle of wholesome ingredients. The village farmers' market became a vibrant hub of activity, with people reveling in the beauty of fresh produce and the knowledge that it could be transformed into something delicious and nourishing.

Join us in the pages that follow, as Emma's culinary odyssey unfolds, sharing not only recipes but also valuable insights, tips, and a roadmap to a healthier, more vibrant you. Just as Emma's village was forever changed by her determination, let this cookbook be your companion on a journey towards a healthier, happier you. May it remind you that every meal is an opportunity to express love for oneself, one's body, and the planet that provides us with the sustenance we need to thrive.

Green Detox Smoothie:

Ingredients:

- 1 cup spinach leaves

- 1/2 cucumber, peeled and chopped

- 1/2 avocado

- 1/2 green apple, cored and diced

- 1/2 lemon, juiced

- 1 cup unsweetened almond milk

- 1 tablespoon chia seeds

- Ice cubes (optional)

Preparation:

1. Place all the ingredients in a blender.

2. Blend until smooth and creamy.

3. Add ice cubes if you prefer a chilled smoothie.

4. Pour into a glass and enjoy this nutritious and refreshing green smoothie.

Grilled Chicken Salad:

Ingredients:

- 4 oz boneless, skinless chicken breast

- 2 cups mixed salad greens (spinach, lettuce, arugula, etc.)

- 1/2 cup cherry tomatoes, halved

- 1/4 cup cucumber, sliced

- 1/4 avocado, sliced

- 1 tablespoon olive oil

- 1 tablespoon balsamic vinegar

- Salt and pepper to taste

Preparation:

1. Preheat your grill or grill pan over medium heat.

2. Season the chicken breast with salt and pepper.

3. Grill the chicken for about 5-6 minutes per side or until fully cooked.

4. Let the chicken rest for a few minutes, then slice it into strips.

5. In a large bowl, combine the salad greens, cherry tomatoes, cucumber, and avocado.

6. Drizzle the olive oil and balsamic vinegar over the salad, and toss to coat.

7. Top the salad with the grilled chicken strips and serve.

Baked Salmon with Lemon and Dill:

Ingredients:

- 4 salmon fillets
- 2 lemons, sliced
- 2 tablespoons fresh dill, chopped
- 2 tablespoons olive oil
- Salt and pepper to taste

Preparation:

1. Preheat the oven to 375°F (190°C).

2. Place the salmon fillets on a baking sheet lined with parchment paper.

3. Drizzle olive oil over the salmon, then season with salt, pepper, and chopped dill.

4. Top each fillet with a couple of lemon slices.

5. Bake in the oven for about 15-20 minutes or until the salmon is cooked through and flaky.

Vegetarian Pad Thai:

Ingredients:

- 8 oz rice noodles
- 1 cup firm tofu, cubed
- 1 cup bean sprouts
- 1 carrot, julienned
- 1 red bell pepper, sliced
- 3 cloves garlic, minced
- 3 tablespoons soy sauce

- 2 tablespoons tamarind paste

- 1 tablespoon brown sugar

- 2 tablespoons vegetable oil

- Chopped peanuts and lime wedges for garnish

Preparation:

1. Cook the rice noodles according to package instructions, then set aside.

2. In a wok or large pan, heat vegetable oil over medium-high heat.

3. Add minced garlic and cook for a minute until fragrant.

4. Add cubed tofu and cook until slightly browned.

5. Add julienned carrots and sliced bell pepper, and stir-fry for a couple of minutes.

6. In a small bowl, mix soy sauce, tamarind paste, and brown sugar. Pour the sauce over the vegetables and tofu in the wok.

7. Add the cooked rice noodles and bean sprouts to the wok, and toss everything

together until well combined and heated through.

8. Serve with chopped peanuts and lime wedges on the side.

Classic Spaghetti Bolognese:

Ingredients:
- 8 oz spaghetti
- 1 lb ground beef
- 1 onion, finely chopped
- 2 garlic cloves, minced
- 1 carrot, grated
- 1 celery stalk, chopped
- 1 can (28 oz) crushed tomatoes
- 1/2 cup beef broth
- 2 tablespoons tomato paste
- 1 teaspoon dried oregano
- 1 teaspoon dried basil
- Salt and pepper to taste
- Grated Parmesan cheese for garnish

Preparation:

1. Cook the spaghetti according to package instructions, then set aside.

2. In a large skillet, brown the ground beef over medium-high heat, breaking it into crumbles as it cooks.

3. Add chopped onions, minced garlic, grated carrot, and chopped celery to the skillet. Cook until the vegetables soften.

4. Stir in crushed tomatoes, beef broth, tomato paste, oregano, basil, salt, and pepper. Simmer for about 20 minutes.

5. Serve the Bolognese sauce over the cooked spaghetti and garnish with grated Parmesan cheese.

Stuffed Bell Peppers:

Ingredients:

- 4 bell peppers (any color)

- 1 lb ground turkey or lean ground beef

- 1 cup cooked quinoa or rice

- 1 cup chopped tomatoes

- 1 cup black beans (canned, drained, and rinsed)

- 1 cup corn kernels (fresh or frozen)

- 1 teaspoon chili powder

- 1 teaspoon cumin

- Salt and pepper to taste

- 1 cup shredded cheddar cheese

Preparation:

1. Preheat the oven to 375°F (190°C).

2. Cut the tops off the bell peppers, remove the seeds, and blanch them in boiling water for about 5 minutes. Drain and set aside.

3. In a skillet over medium heat, cook the ground turkey or beef until no longer pink. Drain excess fat if needed.

4. Stir in chopped tomatoes, cooked quinoa or rice, black beans, corn, chili powder, cumin, salt, and pepper. Cook for a few more minutes until heated through and well combined.

5. Stuff each bell pepper with the filling mixture and place them in a baking dish.

6. Sprinkle shredded cheddar cheese on top of each stuffed pepper.

7. Bake in the oven for about 20-25 minutes or until the peppers are tender and the cheese is melted and bubbly.

Chicken and Broccoli Stir-Fry:

Ingredients:

- 2 boneless, skinless chicken breasts, thinly sliced
- 2 cups broccoli florets
- 1 red bell pepper, sliced
- 1/4 cup soy sauce
- 2 tablespoons oyster sauce
- 1 tablespoon hoisin sauce

- 2 cloves garlic, minced

- 1 tablespoon fresh ginger, grated

- 2 tablespoons vegetable oil

- Cooked rice for serving

Preparation:

1. In a small bowl, mix soy sauce, oyster sauce, and hoisin sauce. Set aside.

2. In a wok or large skillet, heat vegetable oil over medium-high heat.

3. Add minced garlic and grated ginger, and stir-fry for about 30 seconds until fragrant.

4. Add thinly sliced chicken and cook until no longer pink.

5. Toss in broccoli florets and red bell pepper slices, and stir-fry for a few more minutes until the vegetables are tender-crisp.

6. Pour the sauce mixture over the chicken and vegetables, tossing everything together until well coated and heated through.

7. Serve the stir-fry over cooked rice.

Lentil Soup:

Ingredients:

- 1 cup red lentils

- 1 onion, chopped

- 2 carrots, diced

- 2 celery stalks, chopped

- 3 cloves garlic, minced

- 1 can (14 oz) diced tomatoes

- 6 cups vegetable broth

- 1 teaspoon cumin

- 1/2 teaspoon turmeric

- Salt and pepper to taste

- Fresh parsley for garnish

Preparation:

1. Rinse the red lentils thoroughly and set them aside.

2. In a large pot, sauté chopped onions, diced carrots, and chopped celery until they begin to soften.

3. Add the garlic, then heat for an additional minute.

4. Add the vegetable broth, salt, pepper, cumin, turmeric, and diced tomatoes.

5. Bring the soup to a boil, then lower the heat to a simmer, cover, and cook for 15 to 20 minutes, or until the lentils are soft and cooked through.

6. Garnish with fresh parsley before serving.

Caprese Salad:

Ingredients:

- 4 large ripe tomatoes, sliced
- 8 oz fresh mozzarella, sliced
- Fresh basil leaves
- 2 tablespoons balsamic glaze
- 2 tablespoons extra virgin olive oil
- Salt and pepper to taste

Preparation:

1. Arrange the tomato and mozzarella slices on a serving platter, alternating them.

2. Tuck fresh basil leaves between the tomato and mozzarella slices.

3. Drizzle balsamic glaze and extra virgin olive oil over the salad.

4. Season with salt and pepper to taste.

5. Serve as a refreshing appetizer or side dish.

Quinoa and Roasted Vegetable Salad:

Ingredients:

- 1 cup quinoa

- 2 cups mixed vegetables (e.g., bell peppers, zucchini, cherry tomatoes, red onion)

- 2 tablespoons olive oil

- 1 teaspoon dried thyme

- Salt and pepper to taste

- 1/4 cup crumbled feta cheese (optional)

- Fresh parsley for garnish

- Lemon vinaigrette dressing (see below)

Preparation:

1. Preheat the oven to 400°F (200°C).

2. Rinse the quinoa thoroughly in a fine-mesh strainer. In a saucepan, bring 2 cups of water to a boil. Add the quinoa, reduce the heat, cover, and let it simmer for about 15 minutes or until the quinoa is cooked and the water is absorbed.

3. While the quinoa is cooking, prepare the vegetables. Chop them into bite-sized pieces and place them on a baking sheet.

4. Drizzle olive oil over the vegetables, and sprinkle with dried thyme, salt, and pepper. Toss to coat evenly.

5. Roast the vegetables in the preheated oven for about 20-25 minutes or until they are tender and slightly caramelized.

6. Once the quinoa and vegetables are ready, combine them in a large bowl. Optionally, add crumbled feta cheese for extra flavor.

7. Drizzle with lemon vinaigrette dressing (see below) and toss everything together until well combined.

8. Garnish with fresh parsley and serve as a nutritious and satisfying salad.

Lemon Vinaigrette Dressing:

Ingredients:

- 1/4 cup extra virgin olive oil

- 2 tablespoons fresh lemon juice

- 1 teaspoon Dijon mustard

- 1 clove garlic, minced

- Salt and pepper to taste

Preparation:

1. In a small bowl, whisk together the olive oil, lemon juice, Dijon mustard, minced garlic, salt, and pepper until well emulsified.

2. Adjust the seasoning to your taste preferences.

Blueberry Oatmeal Smoothie:

Ingredients:

- 1 cup frozen blueberries

- 1 ripe banana

- 1/2 cup rolled oats

- 1 cup unsweetened almond milk

- 1 tablespoon almond butter

- 1 teaspoon honey (optional)

- Ice cubes (optional)

Preparation:

1. In a blender, combine frozen blueberries, ripe bananas, rolled oats, almond milk, almond butter, and honey (if using).

2. Blend until smooth and creamy.

3. Add ice cubes if you prefer a thicker and colder smoothie.

4. Pour into a glass and enjoy this tasty and filling blueberry oatmeal smoothie.

Grilled Veggie Wrap:

Ingredients:

- 1 large whole wheat tortilla or wrap
- 1/2 cup hummus
- 1 cup mixed grilled vegetables (e.g., eggplant, bell peppers, zucchini, red onion)
- 1/4 cup crumbled feta cheese
- Fresh spinach leaves

Preparation:

1. Warm the whole wheat tortilla slightly, either in the microwave or on a pan.

2. Spread a layer of hummus evenly over the tortilla.

3. Arrange the mixed grilled vegetables on top of the hummus.

4. Sprinkle crumbled feta cheese over the vegetables.

5. Add a handful of fresh spinach leaves on top.

6. Roll up the tortilla tightly into a wrap.

7. Slice in half if desired, and enjoy this flavorful and healthy grilled veggie wrap.

Teriyaki Salmon with Vegetables:

Ingredients:

- 4 salmon fillets

- 1 cup broccoli florets

- 1 cup sliced bell peppers (any color)

- 1/4 cup teriyaki sauce

- 2 tablespoons soy sauce

- 2 tablespoons honey

- 1 tablespoon sesame oil

- Sesame seeds and green onions for garnish

- Cooked rice for serving

Preparation:

1. Preheat the oven to 400°F (200°C).

2. In a small bowl, mix teriyaki sauce, soy sauce, honey, and sesame oil.

3. Place the salmon fillets in a baking dish and pour half of the teriyaki sauce mixture over them.

4. Arrange the broccoli florets and sliced bell peppers around the salmon in the same baking dish.

5. Drizzle the remaining teriyaki sauce mixture over the vegetables.

6. Bake in the oven for about 15-20 minutes or until the salmon is cooked through and the vegetables are tender.

7. Sprinkle sesame seeds and chopped green onions on top before serving over cooked rice.

Black Bean and Corn Salad:

Ingredients:

- 1 can (15 oz) black beans, drained and rinsed
- 1 cup corn kernels (fresh or frozen)
- 1 red bell pepper, diced
- 1/4 cup diced red onion
- 1/4 cup chopped cilantro
- 2 tablespoons lime juice
- 2 tablespoons olive oil
- Salt and pepper to taste
- Avocado slices for garnish

Preparation:

1. In a large bowl, combine black beans, corn kernels, diced red bell pepper, red onion, and chopped cilantro.

2. In a small bowl, whisk together lime juice, olive oil, salt, and pepper to make the dressing.

3. Pour the dressing over the black bean mixture and toss everything together until well combined.

4. Serve chilled and garnish with avocado slices.

Chicken Caesar Salad:

Ingredients:

- 2 boneless, skinless chicken breasts

- 1 head romaine lettuce, chopped

- 1/2 cup croutons

- 1/4 cup grated Parmesan cheese

- Caesar dressing (store-bought or homemade)

- Salt and pepper to taste

Preparation:

1. Season the chicken breasts with salt and pepper.

2. Grill or pan-sear the chicken until fully cooked. Let it rest for a few minutes, then slice it into strips.

3. In a large bowl, combine chopped romaine lettuce, croutons, and grated Parmesan cheese.

4. Drizzle Caesar dressing over the salad and toss everything together until the dressing coats the ingredients evenly.

5. Top the salad with the sliced chicken and serve.

Vegetable Stir-Fried Rice:

Ingredients:

- 2 cups cooked rice (preferably day-old)

- 1 cup mixed vegetables (e.g., peas, carrots, corn)

- 1/2 cup diced tofu or cooked shrimp (optional)

- 2 tablespoons soy sauce

- 1 tablespoon oyster sauce

- 1 tablespoon sesame oil

- 2 cloves garlic, minced

- 2 green onions, sliced

- 2 eggs, lightly beaten

- 2 tablespoons vegetable oil

Preparation:

1. Heat vegetable oil in a wok or large skillet over medium-high heat.

2. Add minced garlic and sliced green onions, and stir-fry for about 30 seconds until fragrant.

3. If using tofu or shrimp, add them to the wok and cook until heated through.

4. Push the ingredients to one side of the wok and pour the beaten eggs onto the space. Scramble the eggs until they are cooked.

5. Add mixed vegetables and cooked rice to the wok, tossing everything together.

6. Mix soy sauce, oyster sauce, and sesame oil in a small bowl, then pour the sauce over the rice and vegetables. Stir-fry for a few more minutes until the ingredients are well combined and heated through.

7. Serve hot as a delicious and filling stir-fried rice dish.

Turkey and Avocado Wrap:

Ingredients:

- 1 large whole wheat tortilla or wrap

- 8 oz sliced turkey breast

- 1 avocado, sliced

- 1/4 cup sliced cucumbers

- 1/4 cup shredded lettuce

- 2 tablespoons Greek yogurt or mayonnaise

- Salt and pepper to taste

Preparation:

1. Lay the whole wheat tortilla flat on a clean surface.

2. Spread Greek yogurt or mayonnaise evenly over the tortilla.

3. Layer sliced turkey breast, avocado slices, sliced cucumbers, and shredded lettuce on top of the sauce.

4. Sprinkle with salt and pepper to taste.

5. Roll up the tortilla tightly into a wrap.

6. Slice in half if desired, and enjoy this healthy and flavorful turkey and avocado wrap.

Ratatouille:

Ingredients:

- 1 eggplant, diced

- 1 zucchini, diced

- 1 yellow squash, diced

- 1 red bell pepper, diced

- 1 onion, chopped

- 3 cloves garlic, minced

- 1 can (14 oz) diced tomatoes

- 2 tablespoons tomato paste

- 1 teaspoon dried thyme

- 1 teaspoon dried oregano

- 2 tablespoons olive oil

- Salt and pepper to taste

- Fresh basil for garnish

Preparation:

1. In a large skillet or pot, heat olive oil over medium heat.

2. Add chopped onion and minced garlic, and sauté until fragrant and slightly softened.

3. Stir in diced eggplant, zucchini, yellow squash, and red bell pepper.

4. Cook for a few minutes until the vegetables start to soften.

5. Add diced tomatoes, tomato paste, dried thyme, dried oregano, salt, and pepper. Stir everything together.

6. Cover the skillet or pot, and let the ratatouille simmer over low heat for about 15-20 minutes until the vegetables are tender.

7. Garnish with fresh basil before serving.

Lemon Herb Grilled Chicken:

Ingredients:

- 4 boneless, skinless chicken breasts

- Zest and juice of 1 lemon

- 2 tablespoons olive oil

- 2 cloves garlic, minced

- 1 teaspoon dried thyme

- 1 teaspoon dried rosemary

- Salt and pepper to taste

Preparation:

1. In a bowl, mix lemon zest, lemon juice, olive oil, minced garlic, dried thyme, dried rosemary, salt, and pepper.

2. Place the chicken breasts in a resealable plastic bag or shallow dish, then pour the marinade over them.

3. Seal the bag or cover the dish, and marinate the chicken in the refrigerator for at least 30 minutes or preferably overnight.

4. Preheat your grill to medium-high heat.

5. Remove the chicken from the marinade and grill each side for about 5-6 minutes or until fully cooked and grill marks appear.

6. Serve the lemon herb grilled chicken with your choice of side dishes.

Pesto Pasta with Cherry Tomatoes:

Ingredients:

- 8 oz pasta of your choice (e.g., penne, fusilli, or spaghetti)

- 1 cup cherry tomatoes, halved

- 1/2 cup homemade or store-bought pesto sauce

- 1/4 cup grated Parmesan cheese

- Fresh basil leaves for garnish

Preparation:

1. Cook the pasta according to package instructions until al dente. Drain and set aside.

2. In a large mixing bowl, combine the cooked pasta, halved cherry tomatoes, and pesto sauce.

3. Toss everything together until the pasta is evenly coated with the pesto and the cherry tomatoes are well distributed.

4. Sprinkle grated Parmesan cheese over the pasta and toss again.

5. Garnish with fresh basil leaves before serving as a tasty and quick pasta dish.

Egg Fried Rice:

Ingredients:

- 2 cups cooked white rice (preferably day-old)
- 2 eggs, lightly beaten
- 1 cup mixed vegetables (e.g., peas, carrots, corn)
- 2 tablespoons soy sauce
- 1 tablespoon oyster sauce
- 2 tablespoons vegetable oil
- Salt and pepper to taste

- Chopped green onions for garnish

Preparation:

1. Heat vegetable oil in a large skillet or wok over medium-high heat.

2. Add the beaten eggs to the skillet and scramble them until cooked.

3. Push the scrambled eggs to one side of the skillet and add the mixed vegetables to the other side. Stir-fry the vegetables until they are heated through and tender.

4. Mix the cooked vegetables and scrambled eggs together in the skillet.

5. Add the cooked white rice to the skillet, breaking up any clumps as you go.

6. Pour soy sauce and oyster sauce over the rice and stir everything together until well combined.

7. Season with salt and pepper to taste.

8. Garnish with chopped green onions and serve this flavorful egg-fried rice.

Tomato and Mozzarella Caprese Chicken:

Ingredients:

- 4 boneless, skinless chicken breasts

- 2 large ripe tomatoes, sliced

- 8 oz fresh mozzarella, sliced

- Fresh basil leaves

- 2 tablespoons balsamic glaze

- 2 tablespoons olive oil

- Salt and pepper to taste

Preparation:

1. Preheat the oven to 400°F (200°C).

2. Season the chicken breasts with salt and pepper.

3. In a skillet over medium-high heat, sear the chicken breasts on both sides until they are golden brown.

4. Transfer the chicken breasts to a baking dish.

5. Top each chicken breast with a couple of tomato slices, fresh mozzarella slices, and fresh basil leaves.

6. Drizzle balsamic glaze and olive oil over the chicken and toppings.

7. Bake in the oven for about 15-20 minutes or until the chicken is cooked through and the cheese is melted and bubbly.

8. Serve the Tomato and Mozzarella Caprese Chicken with your choice of side dishes.

Spinach and Feta Stuffed Chicken:

Ingredients:

- 4 boneless, skinless chicken breasts

- 2 cups fresh baby spinach leaves

- 1/2 cup crumbled feta cheese

- 2 cloves garlic, minced

- 1 tablespoon olive oil

- Salt and pepper to taste

Preparation:

1. Preheat the oven to 375°F (190°C).

2. In a skillet over medium heat, sauté minced garlic in olive oil until fragrant.

3. Add fresh baby spinach leaves to the skillet and cook until they wilt.

4. Remove the skillet from the heat and stir in crumbled feta cheese until well combined.

5. Use a sharp knife to cut a pocket into the side of each chicken breast.

6. Stuff the spinach and feta mixture into the pockets of the chicken breasts.

7. Season the stuffed chicken breasts with salt and pepper.

8. Place the stuffed chicken breasts in a baking dish and bake in the oven for about 20-25 minutes or until the chicken is cooked through and no longer pink.

Grilled Vegetable Quesadillas:

Ingredients:

- 4 large flour tortillas

- 1 zucchini, sliced

- 1 red bell pepper, sliced

- 1 yellow bell pepper, sliced

- 1 red onion, sliced

- 1 cup shredded cheddar cheese

- 2 tablespoons olive oil

- Salt and pepper to taste

- Guacamole and salsa for serving (optional)

Preparation:

1. Preheat your grill or grill pan over medium-high heat.

2. In a large bowl, toss the sliced zucchini, red bell pepper, yellow bell pepper, and red onion with olive oil, salt, and pepper.

3. Grill the vegetables for a few minutes on each side until they are tender and have grill marks.

4. Lay a flour tortilla flat and sprinkle shredded cheddar cheese on one half.

5. Add a layer of grilled vegetables on top of the cheese.

6. Fold the tortilla in half to cover the filling.

7. Grill the quesadilla on the preheated grill or grill pan until the cheese melts and the tortilla becomes crispy.

8. Repeat the process for the remaining quesadillas.

9. Cut the quesadillas into wedges and serve with guacamole and salsa if desired.

Stuffed Bell Peppers with Quinoa and Chickpeas:

Ingredients:

- 4 bell peppers (any color)

- 1 cup cooked quinoa

- 1 can (15 oz) chickpeas, drained and rinsed

- 1 cup diced tomatoes

- 1/2 cup diced red onion

- 2 cloves garlic, minced

- 1 teaspoon ground cumin

- 1 teaspoon ground paprika

- Salt and pepper to taste

- Grated cheese for topping (optional)

Preparation:

1. Preheat the oven to 375°F (190°C).

2. Cut the tops off the bell peppers, remove the seeds, and blanch them in boiling water for about 5 minutes. Drain and set aside.

3. In a skillet over medium heat, sauté diced red onion and minced garlic until they become translucent.

4. Stir in cooked quinoa, drained and rinsed chickpeas, diced tomatoes, ground cumin, ground paprika, salt, and pepper. Cook for a few more minutes until everything is heated through and well combined.

5. Stuff each bell pepper with the quinoa and chickpea mixture.

6. Place the stuffed bell peppers in a baking dish and optionally top with grated cheese.

7. Bake in the oven for about 20-25 minutes or until the bell peppers are tender and the filling is hot.

Mango Salsa Chicken:

Ingredients:

- 4 boneless, skinless chicken breasts

- 1 ripe mango, diced

- 1/2 red bell pepper, diced

- 1/4 cup diced red onion

- 1 jalapeno, seeds removed and finely diced (optional for heat)

- 2 tablespoons fresh lime juice

- 1 tablespoon chopped fresh cilantro

- Salt and pepper to taste

Preparation:

1. Preheat the oven to 375°F (190°C).

2. Season the chicken breasts with salt and pepper.

3. In a small bowl, mix diced mango, diced red bell pepper, diced red onion, finely diced jalapeno (if using), fresh lime juice, chopped fresh cilantro, salt, and pepper.

4. Lay the pre-seasoned chicken breasts in a baking dish.

5. Spoon the mango salsa mixture over the chicken breasts, ensuring it covers them evenly.

6. Cover the baking dish with foil and bake in the preheated oven for about 25-30 minutes or until the chicken is cooked through.

7. Remove the foil during the last 5 minutes of baking to allow the top to brown slightly.

8. Serve the Mango Salsa Chicken with your choice of side dishes for a burst of fresh and tropical flavors.

Greek Chickpea Salad:

Ingredients:

- 1 can (15 oz) chickpeas, drained and rinsed

- 1 cucumber, diced

- 1 cup cherry tomatoes, halved

- 1/4 cup diced red onion

- 1/4 cup chopped Kalamata olives

- 1/4 cup crumbled feta cheese

- 2 tablespoons red wine vinegar

- 2 tablespoons extra virgin olive oil

- 1 teaspoon dried oregano

- Salt and pepper to taste

- Fresh parsley for garnish

Preparation:

1. In a large bowl, combine chickpeas, diced cucumber, halved cherry tomatoes, diced red onion, chopped Kalamata olives, and crumbled feta cheese.

2. In a small bowl, whisk together red wine vinegar, extra virgin olive oil, dried oregano, salt, and pepper to make the dressing.

3. Pour the dressing over the salad and toss everything together until well-coated.

4. Garnish with fresh parsley before serving this light and flavorful Greek Chickpea Salad.

Shrimp and Broccoli Stir-Fry:

Ingredients:
- 1 lb large shrimp, peeled and deveined
- 2 cups broccoli florets
- 1 red bell pepper, sliced
- 3 cloves garlic, minced
- 1 tablespoon grated fresh ginger
- 3 tablespoons soy sauce
- 1 tablespoon hoisin sauce
- 1 tablespoon oyster sauce
- 1 tablespoon sesame oil
- 2 tablespoons vegetable oil
- Cooked rice for serving

Preparation:

1. In a large skillet or wok, heat vegetable oil over medium-high heat.

2. Add minced garlic and grated fresh ginger, and stir-fry for about 30 seconds until fragrant.

3. Add shrimp to the skillet and cook until they turn pink and are fully cooked.

4. Remove the shrimp from the skillet and set them aside.

5. In the same skillet, stir-fry broccoli florets and sliced red bell pepper until they are tender-crisp.

6. Mix soy sauce, hoisin sauce, oyster sauce, and sesame oil in a small bowl, then pour the sauce over the vegetables in the skillet.

7. Return the cooked shrimp to the skillet and toss everything together until well combined and heated through.

8. Serve the Shrimp and Broccoli Stir-Fry over cooked rice.

Mediterranean Quinoa Salad:

Ingredients:

- 1 cup cooked quinoa

- 1 cup diced cucumber

- 1 cup diced tomatoes

- 1/2 cup crumbled feta cheese

- 1/4 cup sliced Kalamata olives

- 1/4 cup diced red onion

- 2 tablespoons chopped fresh parsley

- 2 tablespoons lemon juice

- 2 tablespoons extra virgin olive oil

- Salt and pepper to taste

Preparation:

1. In a large bowl, combine cooked quinoa, diced cucumber, diced tomatoes, crumbled feta cheese, sliced Kalamata olives, diced red onion, and chopped fresh parsley.

2. In a small bowl, whisk together lemon juice, extra virgin olive oil, salt, and pepper to make the dressing.

3. Pour the dressing over the quinoa salad and toss everything together until well-coated.

4. Serve chilled as a refreshing and nutritious Mediterranean Quinoa Salad.

Panko-Crusted Baked Chicken Tenders:

Ingredients:

- 1 lb chicken tenders or chicken breast cut into strips
- 1 cup panko breadcrumbs
- 1/4 cup grated Parmesan cheese
- 1 teaspoon dried Italian seasoning
- 1/2 teaspoon garlic powder
- 1/2 teaspoon onion powder
- Salt and pepper to taste
- 2 eggs, lightly beaten
- Cooking spray

Preparation:

1. Preheat the oven to 400°F (200°C) and line a baking sheet with parchment paper.

2. In a shallow dish, combine panko breadcrumbs, grated Parmesan cheese, dried Italian seasoning, garlic powder, onion powder, salt, and pepper.

3. Dip each chicken tender into the beaten eggs, then coat it with the panko mixture, pressing the breadcrumbs onto the chicken to adhere.

4. Place the coated chicken tenders on the prepared baking sheet.

5. Lightly spray the top of the chicken tenders with cooking spray to promote browning.

6. Bake in the preheated oven for about 15-20 minutes or until the chicken is cooked through and the panko coating is crispy and golden.

7. Serve the Panko-Crusted Baked Chicken Tenders with your favorite dipping sauce.

Veggie Pita Sandwiches:

Ingredients:

- 4 whole wheat pita bread pockets

- 1 cup hummus

- 1 cup shredded lettuce

- 1 cucumber, sliced

- 1 tomato, sliced

- 1/4 cup sliced red onion

- 1/4 cup sliced black olives (optional)

- 1/4 cup crumbled feta cheese (optional)

- Salt and pepper to taste

Preparation:

1. Carefully slice open the pita bread pockets to create a pocket for filling.

2. Spread hummus inside each pita pocket.

3. Stuff the pita pockets with shredded lettuce, cucumber slices, tomato slices, sliced red onion, and sliced black olives (if using).

4. Optionally, sprinkle crumbled feta cheese inside the pita pockets for added flavor.

5. Season with salt and pepper to taste.

6. Serve the Veggie Pita Sandwiches as a quick and nutritious lunch option.

Lemon Herb Roasted Vegetables:

Ingredients:
- 4 cups mixed vegetables (e.g., carrots, bell peppers, zucchini, cauliflower, broccoli)
- 2 tablespoons olive oil
- Zest and juice of 1 lemon
- 1 teaspoon dried thyme
- 1 teaspoon dried rosemary
- Salt and pepper to taste

Preparation:
1. Preheat the oven to 400°F (200°C) and line a baking sheet with parchment paper.
2. In a large bowl, toss mixed vegetables with olive oil, lemon zest, lemon juice, dried thyme,

dried rosemary, salt, and pepper until well coated.

3. Spread the seasoned vegetables in a single layer on the prepared baking sheet.

4. Roast in the preheated oven for about 20-25 minutes or until the vegetables are tender and slightly caramelized.

5. Serve the Lemon Herb Roasted Vegetables as a flavorful and nutritious side dish.

Thai Green Curry with Tofu:

Ingredients:

- 1 block (14 oz) firm tofu, cubed

- 1 can (13.5 oz) coconut milk

- 2 tablespoons Thai green curry paste

- 1 cup mixed vegetables (e.g., bell peppers, bamboo shoots, snow peas)

- 1 tablespoon soy sauce

- 1 tablespoon brown sugar

- 1 tablespoon vegetable oil

- Fresh basil leaves for garnish

- Cooked jasmine rice for serving

Preparation:

1. In a large skillet or wok, heat vegetable oil over medium-high heat.

2. Add cubed tofu and cook until slightly browned.

3. Stir in Thai green curry paste and cook for a minute until fragrant.

4. Pour in the coconut milk and bring it to a simmer.

5. Add mixed vegetables, soy sauce, and brown sugar. Cook until the vegetables are tender-crisp.

6. Serve the Thai Green Curry with Tofu over jasmine rice and garnish with fresh basil leaves.

Italian Sausage and Spinach Pasta:

Ingredients:

- 8 oz penne pasta
- 1 lb Italian sausage links, casings removed and crumbled
- 2 cups fresh baby spinach leaves
- 1 can (14 oz) diced tomatoes
- 1 cup heavy cream
- 1/2 cup grated Parmesan cheese
- 2 cloves garlic, minced
- 2 tablespoons olive oil
- Salt and pepper to taste

Preparation:

1. Cook the penne pasta according to package instructions until al dente. Drain and set aside.
2. In a large skillet, heat olive oil over medium-high heat.
3. Add minced garlic and sauté until fragrant.

4. Add crumbled Italian sausage to the skillet and cook until browned and fully cooked.

5. Stir in diced tomatoes and heavy cream, bringing the mixture to a simmer.

6. Add fresh baby spinach leaves and cook until they wilt.

7. Toss in cooked penne pasta and grated Parmesan cheese, stirring until the pasta is well coated with the sauce.

8. Season with salt and pepper to taste.

9. Serve the Italian Sausage and Spinach Pasta hot.

Orange Glazed Salmon:

Ingredients:

- 4 salmon fillets

- 1/4 cup orange juice

- 2 tablespoons soy sauce

- 2 tablespoons honey

- 1 tablespoon rice vinegar

- 1 teaspoon grated fresh ginger

- 1/2 teaspoon garlic powder

- Salt and pepper to taste

- Sliced green onions for garnish

Preparation:

1. In a bowl, mix orange juice, soy sauce, honey, rice vinegar, grated fresh ginger, garlic powder, salt, and pepper to make the glaze.

2. Preheat your grill or grill pan over medium-high heat.

3. Brush the salmon fillets with the glaze on both sides.

4. Grill the salmon for about 3-4 minutes per side or until it's cooked to your desired level of doneness.

5. Drizzle any remaining glaze over the cooked salmon.

6. Garnish with sliced green onions and serve the Orange Glazed Salmon.

Lentil and Vegetable Soup:

Ingredients:

- 1 cup dried lentils (green or brown), rinsed

- 1 onion, chopped

- 2 carrots, diced

- 2 celery stalks, diced

- 3 cloves garlic, minced

- 1 can (14 oz) diced tomatoes

- 6 cups vegetable broth

- 1 teaspoon dried thyme

- 1 teaspoon dried rosemary

- 1 bay leaf

- 2 tablespoons olive oil

- Salt and pepper to taste

- Fresh parsley for garnish

Preparation:

1. In a large pot, heat olive oil over medium heat.

2. Add chopped onion, diced carrots, and diced celery, and sauté until they start to soften.

3. Stir in minced garlic and cook for another minute until fragrant.

4. Add dried lentils, diced tomatoes, vegetable broth, dried thyme, dried rosemary, and bay leaf to the pot.

5. Bring the soup to a boil, then reduce the heat and let it simmer for about 25-30 minutes or until the lentils are tender.

6. Season with salt and pepper to taste.

7. Garnish with fresh parsley before serving this hearty and comforting Lentil and Vegetable Soup.

Mushroom and Spinach Risotto:

Ingredients:

- 1 cup Arborio rice

- 4 cups vegetable broth

- 1 cup sliced mushrooms (e.g., cremini or button mushrooms)

- 2 cups fresh baby spinach leaves

- 1/2 cup grated Parmesan cheese

- 1/4 cup white wine (optional)

- 2 tablespoons butter

- 1 tablespoon olive oil

- 2 cloves garlic, minced

- Salt and pepper to taste

Preparation:

1. In a saucepan, heat vegetable broth over low heat to keep it warm.

2. In a large skillet, melt butter and olive oil over medium heat.

3. Add minced garlic and sauté until fragrant.

4. Stir in Arborio rice and cook for a minute until lightly toasted.

5. Optionally, pour white wine into the skillet and cook until it is absorbed by the rice.

6. Begin adding warm vegetable broth to the skillet, one ladle at a time, stirring constantly. Allow each ladleful to be absorbed by the rice before adding the next.

7. Continue this process until the rice is creamy and cooked to al dente, usually about 20-25 minutes.

8. In the last few minutes of cooking, stir in sliced mushrooms and fresh baby spinach leaves.

9. Once the risotto is cooked, remove the skillet from the heat and stir in grated Parmesan cheese.

10. Season with salt and pepper to taste.

11. Serve the Mushroom and Spinach Risotto immediately for a satisfying and flavorful dish.

Honey Garlic Baked Salmon:

Ingredients:

- 4 salmon fillets

- 1/4 cup honey

- 2 tablespoons soy sauce

- 2 tablespoons minced garlic

- 1 tablespoon rice vinegar

- 1 tablespoon sesame oil

- Sesame seeds and sliced green onions for garnish
- Cooked quinoa or rice for serving

Preparation:

1. Preheat the oven to 375°F (190°C) and line a baking sheet with parchment paper.

2. In a bowl, mix honey, soy sauce, minced garlic, rice vinegar, and sesame oil to create the marinade.

3. Place the salmon fillets in a shallow dish and pour the marinade over them. Let them marinate for about 15-20 minutes.

4. Transfer the marinated salmon fillets to the prepared baking sheet, reserving the remaining marinade.

5. Bake the salmon in the preheated oven for about 15-18 minutes or until it's cooked to your preferred doneness.

6. Meanwhile, transfer the reserved marinade to a small saucepan and heat it over low heat until it thickens slightly.

7. Drizzle the thickened marinade over the baked salmon.

8. Garnish with sesame seeds and sliced green onions.

9. Serve the Honey Garlic Baked Salmon with your choice of side dishes, such as quinoa or rice.

Vegetarian Stuffed Bell Peppers:

Ingredients:

- 4 large bell peppers (any color)
- 1 cup cooked quinoa
- 1 can (15 oz) black beans, drained and rinsed
- 1 cup diced tomatoes
- 1/2 cup diced red onion
- 1/2 cup diced zucchini
- 1/2 cup corn kernels (fresh or frozen)
- 1 teaspoon ground cumin
- 1 teaspoon chili powder
- Salt and pepper to taste

- Grated cheese (cheddar or pepper jack) for topping (optional)
- Fresh cilantro for garnish

Preparation:

1. Preheat the oven to 375°F (190°C) and grease a baking dish.

2. Cut the tops off the bell peppers and remove the seeds.

3. In a large bowl, mix cooked quinoa, black beans, diced tomatoes, diced red onion, diced zucchini, and corn kernels.

4. Season the mixture with ground cumin, chili powder, salt, and pepper, mixing until well combined.

5. Stuff each bell pepper with the quinoa and vegetable mixture.

6. Optionally, top each stuffed bell pepper with grated cheese.

7. Place the stuffed bell peppers in the greased baking dish and cover them with foil.

8. Bake in the preheated oven for about 25-30 minutes or until the bell peppers are tender and the filling is heated through.

9. Garnish with fresh cilantro before serving the Vegetarian Stuffed Bell Peppers.

Mango Avocado Salad:

Ingredients:

- 2 ripe mangoes, diced

- 1 ripe avocado, diced

- 1/4 cup diced red onion

- 1/4 cup chopped fresh cilantro

- 2 tablespoons lime juice

- 1 tablespoon honey

- Salt and pepper to taste

- Mixed greens for serving

Preparation:

1. In a large bowl, combine diced mangoes, diced avocado, diced red onion, and chopped fresh cilantro.

2. In a small bowl, whisk together lime juice, honey, salt, and pepper to make the dressing.

3. Pour the dressing over the mango and avocado mixture, tossing everything together until well coated.

4. Serve the Mango Avocado Salad over a bed of mixed greens for a refreshing and vibrant side salad.

Lemon Herb Grilled Shrimp:

Ingredients:

- 1 lb large shrimp, peeled and deveined
- Zest and juice of 1 lemon
- 2 tablespoons olive oil
- 2 cloves garlic, minced
- 1 teaspoon dried thyme
- 1 teaspoon dried rosemary

- Salt and pepper to taste

- Skewers for grilling (if using wooden skewers, soak them in water for 30 minutes)

Preparation:

1. In a bowl, mix lemon zest, lemon juice, olive oil, minced garlic, dried thyme, dried rosemary, salt, and pepper to create the marinade.

2. Place the peeled and deveined shrimp in the marinade and toss until coated.

3. Let the shrimp marinate for about 15-20 minutes.

4. Preheat your grill to medium-high heat.

5. Thread the marinated shrimp onto skewers.

6. Grill the shrimp skewers for about 2-3 minutes per side or until they are pink and fully cooked.

7. Serve the Lemon Herb Grilled Shrimp as a flavorful appetizer or main dish.

Veggie Spring Rolls with Peanut Dipping Sauce:

Ingredients:

- Rice paper wrappers

- 2 cups shredded lettuce

- 1 cup shredded carrots

- 1 cup sliced cucumbers

- 1 cup sliced bell peppers (any color)

- 1/2 cup chopped fresh cilantro

- 1/4 cup chopped fresh mint leaves

- 1/4 cup chopped fresh basil leaves

- 1/4 cup chopped roasted peanuts

- 1/4 cup peanut butter

- 2 tablespoons soy sauce

- 1 tablespoon honey

- 1 tablespoon rice vinegar

- 1 tablespoon water

Preparation:

1. Prepare all the veggies and herbs by chopping and shredding them into thin strips.

2. Fill a shallow dish with warm water.

3. Dip a rice paper wrapper into the warm water for a few seconds until it becomes pliable.

4. Place the softened rice paper wrapper on a clean surface.

5. On one end of the rice paper, arrange a small handful of shredded lettuce, shredded carrots, sliced cucumbers, sliced bell peppers, chopped fresh cilantro, fresh mint leaves, and fresh basil leaves.

6. Sprinkle chopped roasted peanuts over the vegetables.

7. Carefully fold in the sides of the rice paper, then roll it up tightly to create a spring roll.

8. Repeat the process to make more spring rolls with the remaining ingredients.

9. In a small bowl, mix peanut butter, soy sauce, honey, rice vinegar, and water to create the peanut dipping sauce.

10. Serve the Veggie Spring Rolls with the Peanut Dipping Sauce for a delicious and healthy appetizer or light meal.

Here are some tips and tricks to help you in your weight loss journey

1. **Set Realistic Goals:** Set achievable and realistic weight loss goals. Gradual and sustainable progress is key to long-term success.

2. **Create a Calorie Deficit:** Consume fewer calories than your body burns to create a calorie deficit and promote weight loss.

3. **Eat a Balanced Diet:** Focus on a balanced diet that includes a variety of fruits, vegetables, lean proteins, whole grains, and healthy fats.

4. **Portion Control:** Be mindful of portion sizes to avoid overeating, and consider using smaller plates and bowls.

5. **Stay Hydrated:** Drink plenty of water throughout the day to stay hydrated and curb unnecessary snacking.

6. **Avoid Sugary Beverages:** Limit or avoid sugary drinks like sodas, energy drinks, and fruit juices as they can be high in calories and low in nutrition.

7. **Incorporate Exercise:** Combine a balanced diet with regular physical activity to enhance weight loss efforts and improve overall health.

8. **Practice Mindful Eating:** Pay attention to your hunger and fullness cues, and eat slowly to savor your food and prevent overeating.

9. **Plan Meals and Snacks:** Plan your meals and snacks ahead of time to avoid impulsive, unhealthy choices.

10. **Avoid Emotional Eating:** Find alternative ways to cope with emotions rather than turning to food for comfort.

11. **Get Enough Sleep:** Aim for 7-9 hours of quality sleep each night as lack of sleep can affect metabolism and appetite regulation.

12. **Reduce Processed Foods:** Minimize processed and high-calorie snacks by opting for whole, nutrient-dense foods.

13. **Keep a Food Journal:** Track what you eat to become more aware of your eating habits and identify areas for improvement.

14. **Incorporate High-Fiber Foods:** Foods high in fiber help you feel full and satisfied for longer periods, aiding in weight loss.

15. **Stay Active Throughout the Day:** Incorporate movement into your daily routine, such as taking short walks, using stairs, or doing household chores.

16. **Find Support:** Join a weight loss group, find a workout buddy, or seek support from family and friends to stay motivated and accountable.

17. **Reward Non-Food Achievements:** Instead of using food as a reward, treat yourself to non-food rewards like a spa day or a new book.

18. **Avoid Skipping Meals:** Skipping meals can lead to overeating later in the day, so prioritize regular, balanced meals.

19. **Practice Portion Control at Restaurants:** When eating out, opt for smaller portions, share dishes, or take leftovers home.

20. **Be Patient and Persistent:** Weight loss takes time, and there may be setbacks along the way. Stay patient and keep persevering toward your goals.

21. **Add Protein to Your Diet:** Including protein in your meals can help increase satiety and prevent muscle loss during weight loss.

22. **Control Stress Levels:** Practice stress-reducing techniques like meditation, yoga, or deep breathing to avoid emotional eating and promote overall well-being.

23. **Limit Alcohol Intake:** Alcoholic beverages are high in calories and can lower inhibitions, leading to overeating. Drink in moderation or choose healthier alternatives.

24. **Eat Mindfully:** Avoid distractions while eating, such as watching TV or using electronic devices, to focus on your meal and enjoy the experience.

25. **Snack Smartly:** Choose healthy and satisfying snacks like fruits, nuts, Greek yogurt, or carrot sticks to keep hunger at bay between meals.

26. **Avoid Late-Night Eating:** Try to finish eating at least 2-3 hours before bedtime to give your body time to digest food properly.

27. **Find Exercise You Enjoy:** Engage in physical activities you enjoy to make staying active feel less like a chore and more like a fun part of your day.

28. **Stay Consistent:** Stick to your weight loss plan consistently, even on weekends or during vacations, to maintain progress.

29. **Keep Healthy Foods Visible:** Store healthier options at eye level in your kitchen, making it easier to reach for nutritious choices.

30. **Stay Educated:** Learn about nutrition and weight loss to make informed decisions about your diet and lifestyle.

31. **Focus on Non-Scale Victories:** Celebrate non-scale victories, such as increased energy, improved sleep, or enhanced physical fitness, in addition to weight loss.

32. **Meal Prep:** Prepare meals and snacks in advance to avoid last-minute unhealthy choices when hunger strikes.

33. **Stay Hydrated with Water-Rich Foods:** Include water-rich foods like cucumbers, watermelon, and celery to increase hydration and help with weight loss.

34. **Eat Whole Fruits Instead of Juice:** Opt for whole fruits over fruit juices, as whole fruits contain fiber that aids in satiety.

35. **Monitor Your Progress:** Keep track of your weight loss progress through weekly weigh-ins or measurements to stay motivated.

36. **Avoid Strict Diets:** Avoid crash diets or extreme restrictions that may lead to nutrient deficiencies and unhealthy eating patterns.

37. **Eat Breakfast:** Start your day with a balanced breakfast to kickstart your metabolism and prevent overeating later in the day.

38. **Try Intermittent Fasting:** Consider intermittent fasting as an eating pattern to help with weight loss and improve metabolic health.

39. **Brush Your Teeth After Meals:** Brushing your teeth after eating can signal the end of eating, reducing the likelihood of unnecessary snacking.

40. **Be Kind to Yourself:** Focus on progress rather than perfection and practice self-compassion throughout your weight loss journey.

Remember, successful weight loss is about making sustainable lifestyle changes that you can maintain in the long term. It's essential to find a balance that works for you and supports your overall health and well-being. If you encounter challenges, don't be discouraged; use them as learning opportunities and keep moving forward. Always consult with a healthcare professional before making significant changes to your diet or exercise routine.

CONCLUSION

In closing, as you turn the final pages of "The Weight Loss Cookbook and Guide," we hope you've embarked on a transformative journey that goes beyond just recipes. Throughout these chapters, we've sought to inspire a profound shift in the way you approach food, health, and self-care. Emma's story, intertwined with her culinary creations, has illuminated the path to a healthier, more balanced life—one that embraces both nourishment and pleasure.

Remember that this journey is not about quick fixes or rigid rules. It's about cultivating a sustainable and meaningful relationship with food. The recipes within these pages are tools for exploration, encouraging you to experiment with flavors, ingredients, and techniques that resonate with your personal preferences and needs. From hearty breakfasts to satisfying dinners, from snacks to desserts, these recipes are designed to make your culinary experience a delightful and healthful adventure.

As you transition to this new way of eating, keep in mind that small changes can yield significant results. Embrace the art of mindful eating—savor each bite, appreciate the textures, and let your senses guide you. Listen to your body's signals of hunger and fullness, allowing it to become your ultimate guide on this journey.

Beyond the kitchen, prioritize movement and physical activity that brings you joy. Remember that wellness is a holistic endeavor, encompassing not just what you eat, but how you move, rest, and care for your mental well-being. Surround yourself with a supportive community, whether it's friends, family, or fellow health enthusiasts, to share experiences, challenges, and victories along the way.

As you continue down the path of transformation, be patient and compassionate with yourself. There will be moments of progress and setbacks, and both are essential parts of the journey. Embrace the learning process and celebrate the victories—whether they're a drop in the number on the scale, an increase in energy levels, or simply the joy of trying a new recipe.

"The Weight Loss Cookbook and Guide" is not just a collection of recipes—it's an invitation to rewrite your relationship with food, nourishing both body and soul. As you explore these culinary creations, remember that you hold the power to shape your wellness narrative. May your journey be filled with delicious discoveries, self-kindness, and a renewed sense of vitality.

Here's to a healthier, happier you—one meal, one choice, and one step at a time. Thank you for allowing Emma's story and the flavors of these recipes to be a part of your voyage toward a brighter and more vibrant future.

Happy Cooking!!!